THE BIBLE CURE

FOR
PROSTATE DISORDERS

DON COLBERT, M.D.

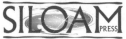

SILOAM PRESS

Living in Health—Body, Mind and Spirit

THE BIBLE CURE FOR PROSTATE DISORDERS
by Don Colbert, M.D.
Published by Siloam Press
A part of Strang Communications Company
600 Rinehart Road
Lake Mary, Florida 32746
www.siloampress.com

Unless otherwise noted, all Scripture quotations are
from Holy Bible, New Living Translation, copyright
© 1996. Used by permission of Tyndale House
Publishers, Inc., Wheaton, IL 60189. All rights
reserved.

Scripture quotations marked KJV are from the King
James Version of the Bible.

Scripture quotations marked NAS are from the New
American Standard Bible. Copyright © 1960, 1962,
1963, 1968, 1971, 1972, 1973, 1975, 1977 by the
Lockman Foundation. Used by permission.
(www.Lockman.org)

Copyright © 2002 by Don Colbert, M.D.

Library of Congress Catalog Card Number: 2002101780
International Standard Book Number: 0-88419-828-6

This book is not intended to provide medical advice or to take the place of medical advice and treatment from your personal physician. Readers are advised to consult their own doctors or other qualified health professionals regarding the treatment of their medical problems. Neither the publisher nor the author takes any responsibility for any possible consequences from any treatment, action or application of medicine, supplement, herb or preparation to any person reading or following the information in this book. If readers are taking prescription medications, they should consult with their physicians and not take themselves off of medicines to start supplementation without the proper supervision of a physician.

02 03 04 05   87654321
Printed in the United States of America

Power Over
Prostrate Disorders

If you are battling disease in your body, you are in a war. Every successful general will tell you that winning a war requires developing a powerful strategy to defeat your enemies. The Bible says, "Prepare plans by consultation, and make war by wise guidance" (Prov. 20:18, NAS).

God's wisdom is vital for you in developing a strategy to fight your enemy—your prostate disorder. Just as a war is fought using various key forces to attack the enemy on different fronts, such as the land, air and sea, so it is with your spiritual battle against disease. You must be prepared to defeat your enemy on every front.

That's why this Bible Cure booklet for prostate disorders involves a natural strategic plan to combat your disease with nutrition, exercise and supplements. In addition, the spiritual strategy will help you to conquer prostate disease in your body through the power of faith and godly wisdom.

More importantly, although God is a healer and strongly desires to cure all of your diseases, He actually prefers for you to experience something even better. God wants you never to get sick! I call that walking in divine health.

The Bible says, "If you will give earnest heed to the voice of the LORD your God, and do what is right in His sight, and give ear to His commandments, and keep all His statutes, I will put none of the diseases on you which I have put on the Egyptians; for I, the LORD, am your healer" (Exod. 15:26, NAS).

In this bold declaration to His people, God strongly urged them to follow His advice. If they did, they could live disease free. Interestingly, as a footnote He added a little about Himself: "I, the Lord, am your healer." God desired their health, and He revealed that desire in outlining lifestyle principles that would keep them healthy.

The Power of Prevention and Prostate Disorders

For men, understanding prevention and implementing the power of prevention in matters of prostate health are vitally important. Most men ignore their prostate glands until they experience minor problems, for example, with an enlarged prostate (called benign prostatic hypertrophy).

Left untreated, however, minor prostate problems may eventually lead to impotence, cancer and death.

If you or someone you know is experiencing a prostate disorder, I have good news. Through lifestyle choices, early detection and treatment options you may prevent the serious consequences of prostate disease or reverse the disease process if it has already begun.

By picking up this Bible Cure booklet, you have taken an exciting first step toward successfully implementing this powerful strategy for prostate health. If you are experiencing prostate disease or cancer, you may be confronting some of the greatest challenges of your life. But with fresh wisdom about God's powerful principles of health and insight into God's power to heal, you can rise to meet the challenge and conquer it.

God revealed His divine will for you through the apostle John, who wrote, "Dear friend, I am praying that all is well with you and that your body is as healthy as I know your soul is" (3 John 2).

With God's help, you can fight back and win. So, as you begin to read through the pages of this booklet, which is filled with hope and encouragement, get ready to become armed with a powerful strategy for prevention and healing! In this book, you will

uncover God's divine plan of health
for body, soul and spirit
through modern medicine,
good nutrition,
and the medicinal power of
Scripture and prayer.

Key Scripture passages throughout this book will help you focus on the power of God. These divine promises will empower your prayers and redirect your thoughts to line up with God's plan of divine health for you—a plan that includes victory over prostate disorders and their destructive physical and emotional effects.

You will gain a strategic plan for divine health in the following chapters:

It is my prayer that these powerful strategies will bring health, wholeness and spiritual refreshing to you—body, mind and spirit. May they deepen your fellowship with God and strengthen your ability to worship and serve Him.

—DON COLBERT, M.D.

A BIBLE CURE PRAYER
FOR YOU

Dear heavenly Father, I thank You that You have provided powerful principles with the promise that if I follow them, You will help me to live disease free. Please provide the grace to help me learn and follow Your principles of prevention and healing. I thank You that it is not Your desire that I would suffer the debilitating physical and emotional effects of prostate disease. As I read through this Bible Cure booklet, give me a special grace to rise up to a bold new level of faith in You. Thank You for making it possible for me to walk in Your divine health for my total being—body, mind and spirit. In Jesus' name, amen.

Chapter 1

Gaining Ground Through Understanding

Gaining a godly understanding is a dynamic first step in accessing the power of prevention. For the Bible says, "Understanding is a fountain of life to him who has it" (Prov. 16:22, NAS).

One powerful method of gaining wisdom is to know your enemy. Therefore, the first step in beating prostate disorders is gaining a good understanding about them.

It takes wisdom to win a war against a powerful foe. The Bible says, "A wise man scales the city of the mighty, and brings down the stronghold in which they trust" (Prov. 21:22, NAS.)

Understanding the Prostate

The prostate is a walnut-shaped gland in men that is about one and a half inches long. It produces most of the fluid that makes up semen—the fluid essential to reproduction.

The prostate lies directly under the bladder and surrounds the upper portion of the urethra, a tube through which urine flows out of the body.

The prostate looks a little like a small doughnut with a straw extending from the center of the doughnut. The straw would be the urethra, which directs urine from the bladder out of the body through the penis.

> *Wisdom is better than weapons of war.*
> —ECCLESIASTES 9:18, NAS

The prostate is positioned in a man's body in front of the rectum and behind the pubic bone. This gland is made of five different parts, which are called zones. We will mention only the two zones that are most problematic: the peripheral zone and the transition zone.

Cancer usually starts in the *peripheral zone,* which contains the majority of glands. Much of this zone can be easily examined during a rectal exam, as this zone is located just adjacent to the rectum. Unfortunately, most men ignore the prostate until it has become diseased or cancer has developed.

The *transition zone* is the area surrounding the urethra. It is here that enlargement usually occurs, signaling the presence of a prostate disorder.

Prostate disorders range from mild to very severe, but most are treatable and highly preventable. The three major prostate disorders can be briefly defined as follows:

1. Prostate cancer

Prostate cancer is often present without any symptoms in its early stages when it's most curable. When symptoms do occur, they are very similar to the symptoms of an enlarged prostate. Unfortunately, at this stage the cancer may have spread to other areas of the body.

2. Enlarged prostate

Also called benign prostatic hypertrophy (BPH), its symptoms are similar to prostatitis, as mentioned below. They include a weak urinary stream, problems starting and stopping urination, excessive nighttime urination and an urgent need to urinate.

3. Prostatitis

Prostatitis most commonly occurs in men between twenty-five and forty-five years of age. Its symptoms include frequent urination, burning while urinating, painful ejaculation, excessive nighttime urination and problems starting and stopping urination.

As we discuss these three problems in more detail, you will be armed with the information you need to help you prevent even minor problems as well as understand the urgency of getting proper treatment if problems do occur.

Prostate Cancer

When it comes to matters of prostate cancer, some men are sitting on a time bomb and don't even know it! In its early stages prostate cancer is often completely curable. But most men never get the needed prostate screening tests to detect this early form of cancer. These preventative tests are the digital rectal exam and the PSA test.

In 1999, 179,300 new cases of prostate cancer were diagnosed, according to the American Cancer Society. Prostate cancer is one of the slowest-growing cancers, which is what makes it so curable through early detection and dietary and lifestyle changes.

The older you get, the greater your risk of developing prostate cancer. The risk of prostate cancer increases with age at an astonishing rate.

A man in his late seventies is one hundred

thirty times more prone to develop prostate cancer than a man in his mid-forties. The risk of developing prostate cancer in men aged forty to forty-nine is one in fifty-three. Astonishingly, it increases to a risk of one in seven for men who are sixty to seventy years old.[1]

By age fifty, nearly one in four men will have some cancer cells in their prostate glands. By the age of eighty, half will have cancer cells.

Prostate cancer is deceptive; it may lie dormant and inconspicuous for decades,

> *Wisdom is better than strength.*
> —ECCLESIASTES 9:16, NAS

only to suddenly start growing and ravage the body with disease. This deceptive nature is why prostate cancer suddenly appears at such an intensified rate in older men. Doubtless it went unnoticed and undetected in their bodies for years.

Early detection can prevent this sudden cancer growth. We can definitely say an ounce of prostate cancer prevention is worth a pound of cure!

Even when prostate cancer does become active, it is still very treatable through surgery and radiation. The cure rate is high in the early stages, but these radical treatments can cause other problems of incontinence or impotence, or both.

These side effects are devastating and depressing, and can make a man feel robbed of his manhood.

Don't Wait!

Since prostate cancer creates no symptoms at all in its early stages, getting screened regularly is a vital strategy in your war against it. Even when prostate cancer is detected, if it is contained to the prostate the cure rate is excellent.

Sadly, however, by the time prostate cancer is finally diagnosed in many men, often it has spread to surrounding tissues, lymph nodes or distant sites. If you are among this group of men, there's still hope. So, don't be discouraged. Read on for a powerful strategy for overcoming even advanced prostate cancer.

The digital rectal exam

If you are forty years of age or older, you should have a yearly digital rectal exam to examine the prostate. If your father, grandfather or other close relatives experienced prostate cancer, you should begin having exams at age thirty-five.

The PSA test

Before getting your PSA tested, abstain from sexual activity for two days prior to the test. In addition, make sure that your physician draws the blood for the PSA before performing the digital rectal exam, since this exam can elevate PSA levels.

Taking certain drugs can affect your PSA score. Propecia, a drug used to treat male-pattern baldness, and Proscar, a drug used in treating an enlarged prostate, can lower your PSA level even if you have cancer. Therefore, be sure to remind your doctor if you are taking either of these drugs.

Are you at a greater risk?

You are at a greater than average risk if you are African American or if you have a family history of prostate cancer.

What Causes Prostate Cancer?

You may wonder why, if God created the incredibly complex natural functions of the prostate, that men are at such a high risk of developing prostate cancer.

Even though we don't know the precise cause of prostate cancer, scientists have learned a great deal about how it develops. In prostate cancer, as with the cells of other cancers, the DNA of the prostate glandular cells has become damaged. DNA is the material that contains your genetic blueprint.

DNA is damaged through an oxidative process involving free radicals. It's not too much different from the oxidative damage seen when iron rusts, when paint flakes or when a sliced apple turns brown. If you were to squeeze lemon juice over an apple slice, it would take much longer to turn brown. That's because the lemon juice contains antioxidants that slow the oxidative process.

Just as a fire burning in a fireplace produces smoke, so your body's cells produce free radicals. Free-radical reactions cause even more free-radical reactions, which can eventually create chain reactions.

Your prostate cell walls are made of fatty acids, and when free-radical reactions occur, these fatty acids become oxidized. Over an extended length of time, with increasing oxidative damage, eventually the nuclei of your cells, where the DNA resides, will sustain damage. When DNA is damaged, the cells may become significantly altered and actually may change into cancer cells.

It has been estimated that nearly every cell in your body takes about ten thousand oxidative hits per day. Imagine someone shooting at you with a BB gun ten thousand times a day. That's similar to what is happening to you at a molecular level.

Initially the fatty cell membranes of the prostate cells take the brunt of the oxidative hits. But over a span of years of this kind of sustained assault, sooner or later the oxidative hits begin to assault the nucleus of the cell, damaging the DNA. The DNA is then altered to produce unhealthy cancer cells.

This cancerous activity is common in the prostate because it tends to be extremely susceptible to oxidative stress and damage. The reason for its susceptibility is the large quantity of the enzyme cyclo-oxygenase the prostate contains. This enzyme produces great amounts of free radicals, which accounts for the high prostate cancer rates in men.

The good news is that this process is very sensitive to dietary changes, which we will see later in this booklet.

Enlarged Prostate or BPH

The second major disorder is an enlarged prostate, called BPH (benign prostatic hypertrophy). It is simply an enlargement of the prostate gland, usually in the area where the prostate surrounds the urethra. Like folding a garden hose in half, this enlargement pinches off the flow of urine, creating an obstruction to the flow. Here are some symptoms:

- Increased frequency in urination
- A weak, dribbly, urinary stream
- Increased nighttime urination
- Problems starting and stopping urination
- An urgency to urinate
- Dribbling at the end of urination

You Are Not Alone

If you are experiencing these problems, you are not alone. As a man ages, generally he experiences the four dreaded characteristics of aging: hair loss, gray hair, wrinkles and an enlarged prostate. Half of all men in their sixties battle BPH, and it affects nearly 80 percent of men in their eighties. That's how common BPH is!

As BPH progresses, it creates a constant feeling of fullness in the bladder because the bladder is never able to completely empty itself. When this happens, men will tend to center their activities around being close to the bathroom because they may need to urinate every hour or so. Can you understand how frustrating this restriction would be to your lifestyle?

Eventually your bladder may be adversely

affected, because it now has to contract more vigorously. Before long it will become thicker and significantly less elastic. When this happens the bladder becomes increasingly less able to hold as much urine, which results in *urge incontinence.* Urge incontinence is when you have a strong urge to urinate but may not make it to the bathroom in time.

If you are experiencing these symptoms, you should understand that they will get increasingly worse and will eventually affect your entire life. You need to contact your primary care physician for a digital rectal exam, a PSA and UA. If your symptoms are severe, consult a urologist.

Take the following quiz to determine the severity of your BPH symptoms.

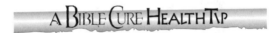

A BIBLE CURE HEALTH TIP

How Do You Rate?

The American Urological Association has devised this worksheet to help doctors evaluate BPH severity. Use the key below to answer the following questions. Write your score on the blank line next to each question.

0=Not at all
1=Less than 1 time in 5

11

2=Less than half the time
3=About half the time
4=More than half the time
5=Almost always

- Over the past month, how often have you had a
  sensation of not emptying your bladder completely
  after you finished urinating?

  0   1   2   3   4   5   _____

- Over the past month, how often have you had to
  urinate again less than 2 hours after you had
  finished urinating?

  0   1   2   3   4   5   _____

- Over the past month, how often have you found
  you stopped and started again several times when
  you urinated?

  0   1   2   3   4   5   _____

- Over the past month, how often have you found it
  is difficult to postpone urination?

  0   1   2   3   4   5   _____

- Over the past month, how often have you had a
  weak urinary stream?

  0   1   2   3   4   5   _____

- Over the past month, how often have you had to
  push or strain to begin urination?

  0   1   2   3   4   5   _____

- Over the past month, how many times did you
  most typically get up to urinate from the time

you went to bed at night until you got up in the
morning?

None 1 Time 2 Times 3 Times 4 Times 5 or more times

0	1	2	3	4	5	_____

TOTAL SCORE _____

Scoring Key

Mild symptoms: 0 to 7 total points
Moderate symptoms: 8 to 19 total points
Severe symptoms: 20 to 35 total points

If you have BPH, even if it's severe or advanced,
there is still much you can do to halt the progression of it. So, don't be discouraged—even if you
scored high on the BPH symptoms test. Just keep
reading!

Prostatitis

The third major prostate condition is prostatitis, a
painful condition involving an inflammation of the
prostate gland. It can be caused by a variety of different things including chlamydia and gonorrhea
infection. Prostatitis can be one of three types:

Acute

Acute prostatitis is an inflammation of the
prostate characterized by discomfort and pain in

prostate characterized by discomfort and pain in the perineal area, frequent urination and, later, retention of urine. Acute prostatitis may cause fever, chills, vomiting, burning during urination, discharge from the penis, painful ejaculation and flu-like symptoms, as well as pain in the lower back and perineum, urinary frequency and a sense of urgency to urinate.

Chronic prostatitis

Chronic prostatitis is an inflammation of the prostate usually causing a dull, aching pain in the lower back and perineum. The symptoms are very similar to chronic bacterial prostatitis.

Chronic bacterial prostatitis

Chronic bacterial prostatitis is an inflammation of the prostate caused by a longstanding bacterial infection. Symptoms include a dull, aching pain in the lower back and perineal region, frequent urination, a burning sensation when urinating, problems starting and stopping urination, decreased urinary stream, painful ejaculation, a sense of urgency to urinate, nighttime urination and occasionally even blood in the semen.

Where Did I Get It?

Both acute and chronic bacterial prostatitis are caused by an infection. Chronic nonbacterial prostatitis is usually related to stress, anxiety, heavy lifting, truck driving, cycling or a number of other activities that tend to irritate the prostate. However, it may also be related to yeast, fungus or another infection.

In addition to treatment by your doctor, several alternative natural treatments that we'll discuss can help

> *O LORD my God, I cried out to you for help, and you restored my health.*
> —PSALM 30:2

you to completely overcome your painful symptoms, reclaim your freedom and regain your health.

Conclusion

Although prostate disorders are a leading cause of pain and early death in men, it doesn't have to be so with you. God has empowered you with life-changing strategies to overcome painful symptoms and live free from disease.

The Bible declares, "The teaching of the wise is a fountain of life, to turn aside from the snares of death" (Prov. 13:14, NAS). Godly wisdom, understanding and courage to face your symptoms and beat them before they progress are keys that can save your life.

Let's pause for a moment and ask God for His help.

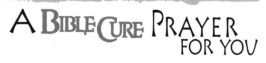

A BIBLE CURE PRAYER
FOR YOU

Dear Jesus, thank You for providing wisdom and power to help me overcome prostate disease and its painful symptoms. I bow my head right now and ask You to be with me in this battle against my prostate disorder. Strengthen my faith, my resolve and my ability to understand and implement Your wisdom and power. Thank You for Your mighty love for me revealed in Your death on the cross. In Jesus' name, amen.

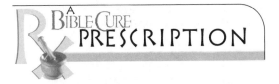

A Bible Cure Prescription for You

Fill in the following scripture verse placing your own name in the blank spaces.

Surely _____ griefs He Himself bore,

And our sorrows He carried;

Yet we ourselves esteemed Him stricken,

Smitten of God, and afflicted.

But He was pierced through for _____
   transgressions,

He was crushed for our iniquities;

The chastening for _____ well-being
   fell upon Him,

And by His scourging _____ is healed.

(ADAPTED FROM ISAIAH 53:4–5, NAS)

Chapter 2

Neutralizing Symptoms Through Nutrition

God's wisdom is vital in developing your strategy to fight your enemy—your prostate disorder—and win. The Bible says, "A wise man is mightier than a strong man, and a man of knowledge is more powerful than a strong man. So don't go to war without wise guidance; victory depends on having many counselors" (Prov. 24:5–6).

Just as a major military action is fought in several strategic theaters at once, so it is with your spiritual battle against disease. You must be prepared to defeat your enemy on every battle front. One of these strategic battle fronts is nutrition.

Just as a nuclear explosion results from the nuclear fission of atoms indiscernible to the naked eye, so tiny changes created in your body through the chemistry of nutrition can powerfully launch you into healing and health.

Nutritional Strategies for Prostate Health

As we have discussed, prostate cancer is a very slowly progressing disease that can lie dormant in the prostate for many years, only suddenly to grow and spread in your latter years. That's why making some relatively minor dietary changes can have a powerfully healing effect—the earlier the better.

As we mentioned in the previous chapter, free radicals are a key factor in the development and progression of prostate cancer.

> The LORD says, "I will guide you along the best pathway for your life. I will advise you and watch over you."
> —PSALM 32:8

That's where diet can have an enormous effect. In addition, if you're experiencing BPH or an enlarged prostate, the following dietary strategies are vital for accessing the power of prevention.

Forgo the Fats

Certain fats generate tremendous amounts of free radicals that feed the dangerous cycle of free radical damage. Epidemiologist Dr. Laurence Kolonel says that men who eat more than 100 grams of fat a day increase their risk of prostate cancer by as much as 50 percent. We have listed below some specific fats to avoid.

Saturated fats

A strong link exists between prostate cancer and a diet high in saturated and polyunsaturated fats. Saturated fats are found in the following:

- Fatty cuts of meats
- Skins of chicken and turkey
- Cheese
- Butter
- Whole milk
- Ice cream
- Fried foods

Linolenic acid

The polyunsaturated fat called *linolenic acid* actually can stimulate cancer cells to grow and metastasize. Linolenic acid is found in the following:

- Soy bean oil
- Safflower oil
- Most other plant oil
- Sunflower oil
- Corn oil
- Fried foods

These fats tend to oxidize very easily, creating tremendous amounts of free radicals that can damage the prostate.

Arachidonic acid

Another polyunsaturated fat called *arachidonic acid* is also associated with an increased risk of prostate cancer. Many researchers believe this fat increases your risk of prostate cancer even more than linolenic acid. Arachidonic acid is found in the following foods:

- Egg yolks
- Red meat
- Cheese
- Whole milk
- Butter
- Ice cream

Alpha-linolenic acid

Alpha-linolenic acid (ALA), believed by researchers to have strong links to prostate cancer, is found in the following foods:

- Red meat
- Margarine
- Walnuts (walnuts are healthy for the heart but high in ALA)
- Mayonnaise
- Vegetable oils (linseed, canola soybean oils)

Fat-Reduction Tactics

Since fats can dramatically increase your chances of getting prostate cancer, here are some fat-reduction principles I recommend:

Reduce red meats

Since these fats tend to promote prostate cancer

in your body, eliminate or reduce your consumption of red meats from your diet. It's best to limit red meats to only 4-ounce servings once or twice a week. I personally eat red meat only about once a month and limit that amount to 4-ounce portions. Choose free-range or kosher poultry and meats.

Reduce milk products

Choose skim milk and skim milk cheeses in place of whole milk and regular cheese. Try replacing regular milk with soy milk as a healthy alternative. This is vitally important for prostate health for two reasons. Number one is the high fat content in milk products, as we've seen. The second extremely important reason is the high calcium content, for excessive calcium intake is linked to prostate cancer, as we will see later.

Forget about fried foods

Fried foods create tremendous free radicals as well as many toxic oxidation products. Peel the skin off of chicken and turkey before eating it, and limit or avoid fried foods.

Limit polyunsaturated fats

Limit or avoid polyunsaturated fats by eliminating most cooking oils (such as sunflower oil, safflower oil and soybean oil), mayonnaise, salad dressings and margarine. Polyunsaturated fats are also found in most snack foods and baked goods.

Limit eggs

Limit your intake of eggs to four per week.

Choose olive oil

Use extra-virgin or virgin olive oil for both cooking and salad dressings. Try extra-virgin olive oil with balsamic vinegar on your salads as a delicious alternative to salad dressings.

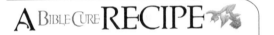

A BIBLE CURE RECIPE

Really Good Salad Dressing

Here's a salad dressing you can make that is really good!

2 Tbsp. extra-virgin olive oil
1 Tbsp. freshly squeezed lemon juice (or apple cider vinegar or balsamic vinegar)
1 Tbsp. purified water
1 tsp. tarragon
1 tsp. garlic salt
1 tsp. parsley flakes
Dash of pepper
Dash of salt

2–3 drops Stevia (sweeten to taste)

Shake in cruet or jar. Pour over salad.

Eat good fats

Good fats include:

- Nuts and seeds, especially almonds and macadamia nuts (easy on the peanuts and cashews)
- Avocados
- Guacamole

Prefer fatty fish

If you are a fisherman and love fish, you're in luck. Fatty fish such as salmon, mackerel, herring and sardines are great for you. Choose fatty fish whenever you can.

Exposure to Certain Chemicals

Farmers tend to have an increased risk of developing prostate cancer, probably due to their exposure to chemicals such as herbicides and pesticides.

Herbicides, pesticides, PCBs, petroleum products and plastics are called xenoestrogens. They are actually synthetic forms of the female hormone estrogen and can mimic the effects of estrogen in you.

Increased amounts of estrogen in men may actually strengthen the prostate-cancer-causing effects of the male hormone testosterone. Testosterone is the primary fuel for prostate cancer, and estrogen can make testosterone more powerful and thus fuel cancer.

You can reduce your exposure to xenoestrogens by including more organic foods and vegetables in your diet. In addition, avoid fatty cuts of meat since this fat is where many of these chemicals are concentrated.

> *The righteous man will flourish like the palm tree, he will grow like the cedar in Lebanon.*
> —PSALM 92:12, NAS

Eating God's Food

Think about eating God's food instead of man's food. What I mean is, try to eat those foods that are more naturally what God created, such as fruits, vegetables and whole, natural grains. Avoid processed and packaged foods, such as TV dinners, white bread, canned vegetables and fruits, sodas, fast foods, cookies, cakes and chips.

Besides decreasing your intake of red meats and fats, increasing the amounts of fruits and vegetables you eat is extremely beneficial. The

National Cancer Institute recommends five to nine servings of fruits and vegetables daily.

Vegetables with powerful anticancer benefits include:

- Broccoli
- Brussels sprouts
- Cabbage
- Cauliflower

These cruciferous vegetables boost the effects of detoxification in the liver, which protect against carcinogens (cancer-causing substances).

Choose fresh vegetables whenever possible over frozen and canned. Fresh broccoli or fresh cabbage are much more effective against cancer than their processed relatives. Brussels sprouts are even better. If you can't get fresh, make frozen your second choice, and avoid canned fruits and vegetables when possible.

The most important of the phytonutrients found in cruciferous vegetables is an indole called DIM. If you just don't like cruciferous vegetables or simply can't get enough of them, you can get the same benefits with a DIM supplement, which we'll discuss later. (Other cruciferous vegetables include kale, collard greens, mustard greens, turnips and radishes.)

Phyto Power!

Some of the most important nutrients for fighting cancer are the phytonutrients. These are simply plant-derived nutrients that contain antioxidants. Many of these are found in colorful pigments of fruits and vegetables, such as the chlorophyll of green vegetables, the carotenes or carotenoids of orange fruits and vegetables and the flavonoids in berries.

Let's take a brief look at some of these fascinating natural healers.

Carotenoids

More than six hundred carotenoids are found in red, orange, yellow and dark green fruits and vegetables. These include:

- Carrots
- Watermelon
- Pink grapefruit
- Sweet potatoes
- Squash
- Tomatoes
- Spinach, kale, collard greens
- Cantaloupe
- Yams

Lycopene

This carotenoid is found in the red pigment of carrots, tomatoes, pink grapefruit and watermelon. This powerhouse reduces the risk of prostate cancer.

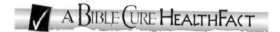

✓ A BIBLE CURE HEALTHFACT

Go Italian!

Do you love spaghetti? A study of forty-eight thousand men over a five-year period found that men who ate ten servings or more of tomato-based products, which contain lycopene, had a 35 percent lower risk of prostate cancer than men who ate less than 1.5 servings a week.

When tomatoes are cooked, as in tomato sauce, they release more lycopene into your system than when you eat fresh tomatoes. So start eating more tomato-based products such as spaghetti sauce, marinara sauce and tomato soup. Just skip the meatballs.

HEALTHFACT HEALTHFACT HEALTHFACT HEALTHFACT HEALTHFACT HEALTHFACT HEALTHFACT

Phytonutrients are powerful nutrients for cancer prevention. Your grandmother probably told you to eat a colorful array of various fruits and vegetables, and you may have thought she was reciting another homespun wife's tale. But she was right—even if she didn't know why.

Made in America

Preferring to have your clothes and cars made in America is good, but that is not true of your American diet. The most common foods eaten in America are white bread, coffee, hot dogs and junk food. All of these are very bad for your health, especially for the health of your prostate. Believe it or not, the average American eats over seven hundred donuts a year. If you are an average American in respect to your diet, you are digging your own grave with your fork.

Lighten Up on Sugar

Believe it or not, cancer actually feeds on the sugar in your body. That's why you should limit your intake of sugar and other high-glycemic starchy foods, such as white bread, white rice, pasta and others.

In addition, eating sugary foods, starches and refined carbohydrates raises your insulin levels. Insulin is another growth factor for the prostate cells and may trigger rapid growth of the cancer cells. For more information on lowering your blood insulin level, see my books *The Bible Cure for Diabetes* and *The Bible Cure for Weight Loss and Muscle Gain*.

Fantastic Fiber

Another primary nutritional key for beating prostate cancer is fiber. The National Cancer Institute recommends getting 25–30 grams of fiber daily. Most Americans don't get nearly this much. To increase fiber in your diet, eat more of the following foods:

- Beans
- Fruits (pears, apples, oranges)
- Oat bran
- Peas
- Psyllium
- Rice bran
- Ground flax seeds
- Other kinds of soluble fiber

Soluble fiber lowers testosterone levels by increasing the excretion of testosterone in the feces.

One word of caution, however; if you increase your intake of beans, start slowly and supplement with Beano, which contains an enzyme that will help digestion.

The Power of Green Tea

Green tea is another powerful antioxidant. It is high in phytonutrient polyphenols called catechins. The catechin EGCG is one of the most powerful antioxidants known to man.

It's actually believed that EGCG in green tea inhibits enzymes necessary for the growth of cancer. Three cups of green tea daily are enough to inhibit cancer growth. Black tea, which is more common in the U.S., may also work as well as green tea.

When you drink tea, don't use sugar or sweeteners. Try using liquid Stevia, an herbal sweetener that contains no cancer-causing chemicals.

Sensational Soy

Foods made with soy are vital for preventing prostate cancer. That's because soy contains certain phytonutrients called isoflavones that help reduce the impact of both sex hormones, estrogen and testosterone. Also, if you already have prostate cancer, soy will help reduce the risk of it spreading.

The ingredient in soy that provides this powerful effect is called genistein. It is the most powerful isoflavone for protecting against prostate cancer. Genistein has approximately $\frac{1}{1000}$ the strength of estrogen and also acts as an antioxidant.

In addition, genistein also helps block angiogenesis, which is the growth of new blood vessels by a cancerous tumor. In other words, it helps to prevent the spread of prostate cancer.

The Asian Experience

Chinese and Japanese men have 90 percent less risk of prostate cancer. The reason is that their diets are filled with soy products, very little meat and very few bad fats.

When Japanese and Chinese men move to America and start eating the American diet, their rate of developing

> *The LORD saves the godly; he is their fortress in times of trouble.*
> —PSALM 37:39

prostate cancer increases dramatically, according to epidemiologist Laurence Kolonel, M.D., Ph.D. In addition, their children and grandchildren have an even greater risk.

The typical Japanese diet contains soy, rice, veggies and fish. Compare that to the standard American diet, which is high in fat, sugar, meat, dairy, fried foods, processed foods and fast foods.

Most American men only eat 1 to 3 milligrams of isoflavones per day, while the average Japanese man eats approximately 12 milligrams per day.

Mike Milken, founder of the Association for the Cure of Cancer of the Prostate, recommends boosting your intake of soy protein to 40 grams per day. In a study of men's dietary habits in forty-two different countries, Dr. J. R. Herbert of the University of Massachusetts Medical School found that eating soy was four times as effective in reducing the risk of prostate cancer as any other dietary factor.[1]

Soy Solutions

That's powerful information! But how can you increase soy in your American diet? Here are some good suggestions:

Begin substituting regular milk, which is high in calcium, with soy milk. For many American men this is a difficult adjustment. However, new research reveals that men who consume more than 2000 milligrams of calcium a day have three times the risk of getting advanced cancer of the prostate as compared to men whose calcium intake is less than 500 milligrams of calcium a day.

If your taste buds balk at the change from cow's milk to soy milk, don't worry. There are many other soy solutions to add to your diet. Here are a few more:

- Use soy cheese instead of regular cheese.
- Drink soy shakes for breakfast (see the recipe below).

- Eat soy nuts.
- Use tempeh, tofu or soy flour.
- Eat soy burgers, not regular hamburgers.

Genistein is the most powerful phytonutrient in soy. I recommend at least 20 milligrams two times a day.

As a precaution, avoid soybean oil because it actually is considered a bad oil. Also, use soy sauce sparingly because it is high in salt and low in phytonutrients.

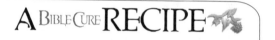

A BIBLE CURE RECIPE

A Sensational Soy Shake

You can make a delicious soy shake to help you increase your daily intake of soy. Mix together the following ingredients in a blender:

> 1 cup of soy milk
> 1–2 Tbsp. of soy protein powder
> ¼ to ½ cup fresh or frozen blueberries,
>   strawberries (or any other berries)
> 5 ice cubes (optional)

Add a small amount of Stevia to sweeten to taste Blend until smooth.

Wet Your Whistle, Partner!

Besides plenty of good, healthy, colorful "God's food," you also need to keep your whistle good and wet all day long with plenty of filtered water. Don't go through a day without drinking at least two to three quarts of filtered water. Water is essential to the health of your prostate and to your overall health, too.

Don't Deny Yourself Dessert

For dessert, try eating fresh fruits and fruit salads. Before long you'll wonder why you liked the sweets so much. Still, you may have a small slice of cake (without the gooey, white icing, of course) once in a while. In moderation, a little treat for special occasions never hurts.

Special Dietary Strategies for Prostatitis

If you are suffering with acute or chronic bacterial prostatitis, your doctor will prescribe antibiotics. Although these powerful drugs truly are modern wonders, they are not harmless. Antibiotics are the first line of treatment for prostatitis. However, it usually takes weeks to months to cure the infection. Unfortunately, some patients continue to have recurring bouts of chronic prostatitis. If you continue having repeated bouts of prostatitis, I recommend boosting your immune system by taking the specific supplements for this problem you will find in the next chapter on supplements.

Antibiotics can create havoc in your body, disrupting the delicate balance of flora in your

> *This I know, that*
> *God is for me.*
> —PSALM 56:9, NAS

intestinal tract. Therefore, it's essential that when you take antibiotics for the extended time span required to eradicate certain types of prostatitis, you also must adhere to a dietary strategy to prevent serious side effects.

If you are taking antibiotics, I strongly urge you to go on the candida diet for the duration of your treatment. You can find an expanded version of this diet in *The Bible Cure for Candida and Yeast Infections.*

Candida and Your Sweet Tooth

Sugar-rich foods are the single most important contributing factor to candida overgrowth. That's why sugar must be strictly avoided for a season of time so that your body has a chance to reclaim its natural balance.

Even the sugars found in fruit juices and high-sugar vegetable juices like carrot juice must be omitted as well as some fruits while you are on the candida diet.

A BIBLE CURE HEALTH TIP

Here's a candida diet checklist that provides the basic foods to avoid until your body recovers. Candida feeds on certain foods, and these foods will need to be eliminated for a season.

Check the foods you will stop eating until your body's balance is restored.

- ❑ No sugar of any kind—white sugar, brown sugar, honey, molasses, barley, malt, rice syrup, etc.
- ❑ No artificial sweeteners—Sweet 'N Low, Nutra-Sweet, Equal, etc. (Stevia is allowed.)
- ❑ No fruit juice of any kind for the first three months, then gradually added back into diet if tolerated.
- ❑ No fruit of any kind for the first three weeks, then gradually added back into diet starting with low-glycemic fruits such as apples, kiwi, berries, grapefruit, lemons and limes.
- ❑ No dairy food of any kind—milk, cheese, cottage cheese, ice cream, sour cream, etc. (A small amount of organic butter and yogurt and

kefir with no lactose, sugar or fruit are acceptable.)

❑ No gluten grains of any kind found in wheat, rye, white or pumpernickel breads, or found in pastry, crackers, etc. (Brown rice bread found in the frozen section of the health food store is a good replacement. Millet bread is also acceptable.) Oats contain less gluten, however, and may not be tolerated by those with severe candida.

❑ No breads or other foods containing yeast

❑ No alcoholic beverages of any kind

❑ No dry roasted nuts (Nuts in the shell—other than peanuts or cashews—are acceptable. The shell protects them from molding.)

❑ No vinegar and vinegar-containing foods with the possible exception of raw, unfiltered apple cider vinegar in those with mild candida

❑ No soy sauce, tamari or natural root beer

❑ No vitamin and mineral supplements containing yeast

❑ No pickled foods or smoked, dried or cured meats, including bacon

❑ No deep-fried foods of any kind

❑ No mushrooms

A Final Word About Prostatitis

Many men find the symptoms of chronic non-bacterial prostatitis are relieved by doing nothing more than eliminating alcohol, caffeine and spicy food from their diets. So, if you have minor symptoms of prostatitis, carefully consider how your diet may be affecting you. You may be sensitive or allergic to a particular food, such as chocolate, dairy products, eggs, wheat, corn, soy or yeast. Believe it or not, the very foods you crave may be the ones causing you problems. Relief for chronic prostatitis may be as simple as eliminating the offending food or foods from your diet. For more information about what foods may be causing your body to react, see *The Bible Cure for Allergies*.

Conclusion

Don't be complacent about prostate disease. You can prevent it or turn it around as you seek wise, godly counsel regarding your health. The Bible promises that "the words of the wise bring healing" (Prov. 12:18).

Remember, if you are battling a prostate disorder, you are in a war. Once again, the Bible states, "Don't go to war without wise guidance;

victory depends on having many counselors" (Prov. 24:6). God is on your side, and, therefore, I know you will win!

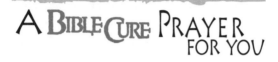

A BIBLE CURE PRAYER
FOR YOU

Dear God, thank You for caring deeply for my health and for providing a sound, godly strategy for me to overcome prostate disease. Help me to change my dietary habits to strengthen my body against this disease. I know You desire health for me—body, mind and spirit. As I access Your strategies for health, help me to come to know You better as the healer of both my body and my soul. In Jesus' name, amen.

R_A BIBLE CURE PRESCRIPTION

Check the dietary changes you are willing to make to prevent or reverse the progression of prostate disease.

- ❏ Limit red meats
- ❏ Increase tomato-based foods
- ❏ Limit fried foods
- ❏ Use olive oil
- ❏ Use skim milk products
- ❏ Limit polyunsaturated fats

List the types of fatty fish you will be willing to eat at least once or twice a week.

_____

List the vegetables you like that you will be willing to eat more often.

_____

What types of soy products are you willing to try?

_____

What favorite foods do you need to limit, avoid or substitute to conquer prostate disease?

_____

_____

Chapter 3

Seizing Power Through Supplements

King David well understood what it meant to go into battle against a formidable enemy. He was a warrior king who sought God for many winning strategies against his enemies. He gave God the praise for his victories, declaring on one occasion, "You have armed me with strength for the battle; you have subdued my enemies under my feet" (Ps. 18:39).

If you are battling prostate disease, you too are in a war with a dangerous enemy. Though you are not at war against flesh and blood warriors, your foe is as insidious and destructive as any armed enemy in combat. And just as King David won his battles through strategies he received from God, you too can receive divine wisdom and power against your enemy.

The third strategy of this fivefold Bible cure for

prostate disease cannot unfold without pursuing the first the two strategies we discussed: gaining understanding and combating the disease with good nutrition. Once these strategies are in place, this next strategy involves a power-packed source of metabolic ammunition to defeat disease in your body. This power-packed ammunition is the proper use of supplements.

Supplement Power

Supplements can arm your body with what it needs for a frontal attack against the source of prostate cancer and disease. Taking the right supplements can help you to reduce dramatically your risk of developing prostate disease. Additionally, supplements have the ability to assist your body's battle in reversing prostate disease even after it is diagnosed.

Antioxidant Ammo Against Cancer

Target cancer-causing free radicals in your body with antioxidant ammunition. Antioxidants are powerfully effective in preventing prostate cancer and keeping it from becoming active and spreading when it resides in a dormant state.

In a Finnish study called the ATBC Trial, men

taking the antioxidant vitamin E experienced a 40 percent decreased death rate from prostate cancer when compared with those who didn't take antioxidants. In addition to that, the men also had a 30 percent decreased risk of being diagnosed with prostate cancer.

Here's a list of some powerful antioxidants and other supplements you should take every day.

Vitamin E

Vitamin E is fat soluble, which means it is particularly effective in reaching fatty tissues like those found in the prostate. Take at least 400 IUs of vitamin E per day, and check the label to be sure it is the alpha-tocopherol or mixed tocopherols variety.

Selenium

This power-packed antioxidant is vital for your cancer-busting arsenal. It has been shown that men who have the lowest levels of selenium in their bloodstream were also 50 percent more likely to develop prostate cancer, whereas those with the highest levels were 50 percent less likely to develop prostate cancer.

Selenium and vitamin E complement each other amazingly well. Together they form a powerful shield of antioxidant protection against prostate cancer.

Take at least 200 micrograms of selenium daily.

Vitamin D

Vitamin D has long been seen as a natural cancer protector. A few years ago, scientists discovered that American men who live in the northern states experienced higher mortality rates from prostate cancer than those from the South. These scientists surmised that the leading factor for this difference was vitamin D because sunlight exposure increases the production of vitamin D in the body. Those men living in the southern states would potentially have greater exposure to sunlight than those living farther north.

In addition, a lack of vitamin D is considered a major reason for the increased rates

> *This I know, that God is for me.*
> —PSALM 56:9, NAS

of prostate cancer among African American men because their darker skin absorbs less sunlight, resulting in lower levels of vitamin D.

The best way to increase your vitamin D is to spend more time out of doors in the sunlight, fifteen to twenty minutes daily at noontime is best. If you're trapped in an office all day, try eating your lunch at a picnic table outdoors.

Adequate amounts of vitamin E, selenium and vitamin D can be found in a comprehensive multivitamin such as Divine Health Multivitamin for Men. (To order, call 407-331-7007.)

Coenzyme Q_{10}

Coenzyme Q_{10} is found in foods such as salmon, liver and organ meat. However, it is very difficult to obtain adequate coenzyme Q_{10} in one's diet. Coenzyme Q_{10} is involved in the production of energy, thus energizing the immune system. It is also a powerful antioxidant, which protects the body from free radicals. It also helps the body regenerate vitamin E so that the vitamin E continues to quench free radicals. I recommend at least 50 milligrams of coenzyme Q_{10} once or twice a day.

Lipoic acid

Lipoic acid is a powerful antioxidant that protects the cells from free-radical assaults in both fat-soluble and water-soluble compartments of the cell. The cell and nuclear membranes are made mainly of fats, and the cell itself is composed of water. Vitamin E, coenzyme Q_{10} and lipoic acid protect the fatty portion of the cell and nuclear membranes from free radicals. Vitamin C and glutathione protect the water portions of the cell. Lipoic acid can recycle the fat-soluble antioxidants (vitamin E and coenzyme Q_{10}) and the water-soluble antioxidants (vitamin C and glutathione). Lipoic acid is a super antioxidant and is essential for any cancer protection plan. I recommend at least 50 milligrams two times a day. Divine Health Advanced Antioxidant contains both coenzyme Q_{10} and lipoic acid. To order this product, you may call 407-331-7007.

Phytonutrient Supplements to Fight Cancer

As we discussed, phytonutrients found in cruciferous vegetables work powerfully to fight against cancer. We mentioned that the most important phytonutrient in cruciferous vegetables is an indole called DIM, which you can take as a supplement if you do not like or cannot eat enough broccoli, cauliflower and other cruciferous vegetables.

Indolplex

Indolplex is a DIM supplement that you can order by calling 800-931-1709. Take 60 milligrams of Indolplex two times a day.

Moducare

Moducare, composed of plant sterols and

sterolins, has dramatic immune-optimizing properties. Studies have shown that it increases natural killer cell activity in vitro. I recommend two tablets two or three times a day one hour before meals on an empty stomach. (To order, call 407-331-7007.)

Supplement Strategies for BPH

In addition to preventing and treating cancer, supplements are a powerful part of your health strategy for BPH or benign prostatic hypertrophy.

Saw palmetto

This powerful prostate-healing herb is made from the berries of the saw palmetto plant, which is found in my home state of Florida. Saw palmetto has been recognized as an effective treatment for BPH in many European countries.

Symptoms of BPH improve in about four to six weeks in two-thirds of men who take saw palmetto. Some studies have shown that saw palmetto is as effective as the medication Proscar, and with far fewer side effects.

The standard dose of saw palmetto is 160 milligrams twice a day. However, you may increase this to 320 milligrams twice a day after six weeks if your symptoms have not improved.

Before you begin taking saw palmetto, it's important to have your doctor give you a digital rectal exam and a PSA test to rule out prostate cancer. In addition, be sure to inform your doctor in future visits that you are taking saw palmetto before having a PSA screening since it may lower your PSA level.

Beta-sitosterol

This is probably the most important supplement you can take for BPH. Beta-sitosterol is a powerful plant nutrient used in Germany for more than twenty years for treating benign prostatic hypertrophy.

Some plants such as rice bran, soybeans and wheat germ contain particularly high levels of beta-sitosterol.

> *No weapon that is formed against thee shall prosper.*
> —Isaiah 54:17, KJV

Sitosterol inhibits the production of inflammatory prostaglandins, which in turn lowers prostate congestion.

Moducare contains beta-sitosterol as well as other sterols and sterolins. I recommend two tablets of Moducare two to three times a day one hour before meals on an empty stomach. Even with this amount, it may take months to experience relief from your symptoms. (To order, call 407-331-7007.)

Pygeum Africanum

Another powerful herb that improves the symptoms of BPH is *Pygeum Africanum,* made from an evergreen tree that is native to Africa. The bark contains active sterols and fatty acids, and *Pygeum Africanum* actually contains beta-sitosterol. However, studies indicate that saw palmetto is more effective than *Pygeum Africanum.*

The standard dosage of *Pygeum Africanum* is 100 milligrams of the standardized extract twice a day.

Nettle root

Another herb effective in the treatment of BPH is nettle root. This herb is often combined with saw palmetto and *Pygeum Africanum* to treat BPH.

Take 120 milligrams twice a day.

Zinc

Getting enough zinc is vital for prostate health, especially if you have BPH. Prostate secretions contain high concentrations of zinc. Therefore, zinc plays an important role in healthy prostate functioning.

A simple screening test to help determine if you possibly are deficient in zinc is the zinc tally test. Place a teaspoon of zinc sulfate on your tongue, and hold it in your mouth for five seconds. If you do not taste the zinc, which has a bitter flavor, then you are probably lacking zinc.

Take 45 to 60 milligrams of zinc in tablet form daily. Repeat the zinc tally test after a month of taking supplements. If you still cannot taste the zinc, then you are probably not absorbing enough of it into your system. You may need to try a liquid form of this supplement.

Divine Health Prostate Support

I call this supplement the Michael Jordan of prostate supplements. It can do a slam-dunk against prostate disease like no other in its league. Take this excellent supplement for BPH. It contains phytosterols, saw palmetto, *Pygeum Africanum,* nettle root and selenium. It also contains zinc. You can obtain this supplement by calling 407-331-7007.

Take one capsule two times a day.

Bullets for Chronic Prostatitis

Selenium

For chronic prostatitis, you don't want a cap

gun. You need supplement power that packs a big bang. Boost your immune system against this chronic problem with the power of selenium. Take 200 micrograms of selenium two times a day for chronic cases of prostatitis.

Olive leaf extract

I also recommend olive leaf extract for its effectiveness against most viruses and bacteria. Take 500 milligrams three times per day.

Immuni-T

Immuni-T is a comprehensive product containing mushroom extracts and more than twelve active ingredients to support the immune system. If you have chronic prostatitis, take one to two tablets two times per day. You can order this product by calling 800-580-PLUS.

A Rule of Thumb

If this seems like a long list of supplements, let me provide an easy-to-follow guide for you.

For cancer prevention use:

- Vitamin E, 400 IU a day
- Selenium, 200 mcg. a day
- Vitamin D, 400 IU a day

- Vitamin C, 250 mg. three times a day (as an antioxidant)
- Lipoic acid, 50 mg. two times a day (as an antioxidant)
- Coenzyme Q_{10}, 50 mg. two times a day (as an antioxidant)
- DIM (Indolplex), 60 mg. two times a day
- Lycopene, 10 to 15 mg. a day
- Moducare, two tablets two times a day
- Genistein at least 20 mg. two times a day

You can obtain vitamins E, D, C and selenium by taking a comprehensive multivitamin such as Divine Health's Multivitamin for Men. Coenzyme Q_{10} and lipoic acid are found in Divine Health's Advanced Antioxidant.

If your PSA is elevated and your doctor suspects that you have cancer cells or cancer in a dormant state:

- Take the same list of supplements as above.
- Increase Moducare to three tablets three times a day one hour before meals
- Take MGN-3, 500 mg. three times a day (may be obtained from a health food store).

For BPH prevention, take:

- Divine Health Prostate Support, one tablet two times a day
- Comprehensive multivitamin (as directed)

If you are experiencing mild to moderate BPH, take:

- Divine Health Prostate Support, one tablet two times a day
- Comprehensive multivitamin (as directed)
- Moducare, two tablets three times a day one hour before meals

If you are experiencing severe BPH:

- Consult with a urologist.
- Take the above dosages of Divine Health Prostate support and a multivitamin (as directed).
- Increase Moducare to three tablets three times a day one hour before meals.

Avoid Supplemental Hormones

If you are at a high risk for developing prostate cancer, avoid all supplemental hormones, including testosterone, androstenedione and DHEA.

These supplemental hormones can actually

promote the development of prostate cancer in some men.

Conclusion

I hope you've learned by now that you are not hopeless or helpless. Using a powerful natural and spiritual strategy you can mount an armed resistance that will help to defeat prostate disease in your body forever.

You are in a war for your health. In every war there are generals whose authority governs the actions of his soldiers. My prayer for you is that you might begin to discover Jesus Christ as the most powerful General, whose wisdom and compassion can lead you to advance boldly against every attack. As you acknowledge His authority in your life, you will say with King David, "Blessed be the LORD, my Rock, who trains my hands for war, and my fingers for battle" (Ps. 144:1, NAS).

> *But with us is the LORD our God to help us and to fight our battles.*
> —2 CHRONICLES 32:8, NAS

A BIBLE CURE PRAYER
FOR YOU

Dear Jesus, I thank You that You are a mighty general in this war against the enemy of disease that seeks to attack my body. As a great healer, You have defeated every disease and destroyed all my enemies, whether physical or spiritual. Thank You for providing a powerful strategy that will overcome prostate disease and restore my body to complete health. In Jesus' name, amen.

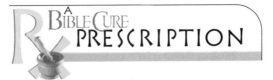

A BIBLE CURE
PRESCRIPTION

From what prostate disorders are you presently suffering?

_____

Do you sense a need to prevent prostate cancer in your body?

_____

Do you have any factors, such as a relative with prostate disease, that predispose you to prostate disease? Describe.

_____

_____

List the supplements that you will be taking for prostate health, and discuss why you plan to take them.

_____

_____

_____

Chapter 4

Energizing Through Exercise, Activities and Treatments

God is a brilliant strategist, a powerful force against an onslaught of overwhelming circumstances. The Bible says, "The LORD is my strength and my song; he has become my victory. He is my God, and I will praise him . . . The LORD is a warrior" (Exod. 15:2–3). God is powerfully active in your warfare against disease in your body.

Let's take a look at active counterattacks to prevent, block and reverse prostate disease in your body.

Beating Cancer With Exercise

A key factor in preventing prostate cancer in your body is to exercise more, especially if you have a desk job or spend a great deal of time driving or sitting. Living under stressful circumstances at work without relieving some of that stress through physical exercise can be disastrous. The risk of prostate cancer was lowered by 50 percent in men over seventy who consistently exercised at high levels.

A regular workout will help your body to release the built-up stress and to condition your body for lifelong health. In contrast, if you have BPH, inactivity may cause your body to retain urine. Even a small amount of exercise can reduce urinary problems caused by an enlarged prostate.

Here are some pointers for working out:

- Choose an activity that you will stick with. Team sports are great as a kind of support group to keep you coming regularly to play with a baseball or basketball team that meets often.
- If you love to golf, be sure to walk and let the older guys have the carts (no matter what your age). Brisk walking will provide the workout you need.
- Exercise for at least twenty minutes per day a minimum of three times per week.

- Check your pulse periodically and exercise within your target heart-rate zone. Find your target range in the following Health Tip.

Your Predicted Heart Rate

Calculate your predicted heart rate using this formula:
220 minus [your age] = _____
x .65 = _____ x .80 = _____
Calculate your target heart zone using this formula:
220 minus [your age] = _____
x .65 = _____
[This is your minimum.]
220 minus [your age] = _____
x .80 = _____
[This is your maximum.]

This example may help: To calculate the target heart zone for a 40-year-old man, subtract the age (40) from 220 (220- 40=180). Multiply 180 by .65, which equals 117. Then multiply 180 by .80, which equals 144. A 40-year-old man's target heart rate zone is 117–144 beats per minute.

Physical Therapy for Prostatitis

If you have been experiencing symptoms of prostatitis, physical therapy can help. Stretching and relaxing the lower pelvic muscles helps to relieve symptoms in some men. Ask your doctor about including a regimen of physical therapy as a part of your treatment.

In addition, you may find that you benefit from heat therapy, which simply involves adding heat to the muscles in the pelvic area to help them relax. You can do this by using a heating pad, a hot water pack or by soaking in a hot tub.

Your doctor also may introduce biofeedback as another helpful method of relaxing the muscles of the perineum and pelvic area. During biofeedback, a trained therapist applies electrodes and other sensors to various parts of your body. The electrodes are attached to a monitor that displays information about your muscle tension, heart rate and blood pressure.

Researchers don't completely understand why physical therapy works for prostatitis. It's believed that tight and irritated muscles can worsen symptoms. Massage is another method of relaxing the muscles.

When NOT to Exercise

Although exercise is almost always beneficial, it can irritate certain prostate conditions. If you have prostatitis, and biking, jogging, or weightlifting worsens the symptoms, then halt that particular form of exercise until your symptoms have cleared up.

If you have prostatitis, heavy lifting while your bladder is full can cause urine to seep into your prostate. So, be sure to empty your bladder before moving furniture, cutting wood or doing other strenuous exercises.

Avoid occupations that cause excessive vibration to the prostate, including operating heavy equipment, truck driving and so forth.

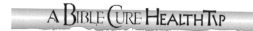

A BIBLE CURE HEALTH TIP

Try These Prostatitis Relief Tips

If you are experiencing chronic nonbacterial prostatitis, try the following to relieve your painful symptoms.

A sitz bath

- Fill a tub with hot, steamy water.
- Dump in 2 cups of Epsom salts.
- Sit in the hot tub with water completely

covering the lower half of your body.

- Relax for fifteen to twenty minutes.
- Repeat twice per day.
- Try adding a few drops of lavender oil to the water for its relaxing effects.

Frequent intercourse

For married men, frequent sexual intercourse will help relieve the symptoms of nonbacterial prostatitis by helping to release the prostatic fluids from the prostate.

Prostate "massage"

Your medical doctor may determine that a prostate massage will help relieve your symptoms by unplugging ducts blocked by bacteria, which allows anti-biotics to penetrate deeper into infected tissues and become more effective. The massage is performed during a digital rectal exam.

Treatment Options

It's important to be aware of your treatment options if you are experiencing a prostate disorder. Let's take a look at some treatment options that will help arm you with wisdom to make winning decisions that can save your life.

Facing a cancer treatment decision

If you've been diagnosed with prostate cancer, consult a urologist and radiation therapist to determine your best options. If your PSA score is between 5 and 10, then the cancer is most likely very localized and treatable. Talk to your urologist before deciding between radiation and surgery.

Total prostatectomy

A total prostatectomy involves the surgical removal of all of your prostate. If you make this difficult decision, be sure that your surgeon is highly skilled in the nerve-sparing prostatectomy procedure. Before you agree to be operated on, ask him how many nerve-sparing prostatectomies he has performed.

Don't neglect to ask him how successful he has been in preventing both impotence and incontinence. Dr. Patrick Walsh at Johns Hopkins Medical Institution is the world's foremost authority on prostate cancer. He has the best results of any other urologist in the world. An astounding 93 percent of his patients have maintained urinary continence, and 86 percent have not become impotent following the procedure.

Other urologists do not have the same expertise or statistical results. Nevertheless, you can find the best surgeon available to you. Look for a urologist who operates at a major medical center and has performed at least one hundred procedures.

Excision by radiation

Radiation therapy for prostate cancer employs radiation to kill cancer cells. Both external beam and seed implants are used. Seed implants are usually radioactive iodine seeds that are metal capsules about ⅕ of an inch long and look like a piece of pencil lead. These seeds are implanted by an ultrasound-guided technique into the area of the prostate cancer. A beam from a large machine positioned over the body delivers external beam radiation.

The most effective results have been obtained by combining these two procedures. Dr. Frank Critz of the Radiotherapy Clinics of Georgia in Atlanta has realized spectacular results in treating over sixteen hundred men with his combined procedure called ProstRcision. In fact, 89 percent of his patients have remained cancer free past the important five- to seven-year benchmark following the treatment. This success rate is unparalleled by any other radiotherapy program.[1]

PC Spes

If you have metastatic prostate cancer, meaning that your cancer has spread beyond the prostate into other parts of your body, take a critical look at a hormonal therapy called PC Spes.

PC Spes is actually a combination of eight different herbs that work similarly to estrogen therapy, which is an excellent therapy for metastatic prostate cancer. DES is the gold standard for estrogen therapy, and PC Spes is considered as effective as DES. PC Spes, however, does have the estrogenic side effects that are unacceptable to many men, such as breast enlargement and decreased sexual desire.

Each of the eight herbs has been shown to have cancer-killing ability while stimulating the immune system to fight cancer, too.[2] Many traditional cancer treatments seriously compromise the immune system. In addition, oral estrogens can increase your risk of developing a heart attack, but PC Spes does not have these risk factors either. It is actually less toxic than aspirin.

> *Cast your burden upon the LORD, and He will sustain you; He will never allow the righteous to be shaken.*
> —PSALM 55:22, NAS

The recommended dosage of PC Spes is three capsules three times a day. You must take this treatment under the close supervision of a doctor even though it is an herbal supplement.

IMPORTANT NOTE: PC Spes should not be taken for localized prostate cancer, but only for metastatic prostate cancer. Your doctor or urologist can order PC Spes by calling 714-524-5533.[3]

Do Not Fear

If you are battling prostate cancer or any other prostate disorder, you don't need to fear. Prostate disease is not only treatable— it's beatable! With this fivefold Bible Cure

> *Though a host encamp against me, my heart will not fear; though war arise against me, in spite of this I shall be confident.*
> —PSALM 27:3, NAS

strategy you can launch an aggressive, powerful counterattack against your enemy from each of these battlefronts. We have discussed the first four powerful weapons in your arsenal: godly wisdom, nutrition, supplements and exercise. The final strategic theater of your warfare is doubtless the most important: your faith.

A BIBLE CURE PRAYER
FOR YOU

Dear God, thank You for providing a powerful strategy to combat my prostate disease on all of its major fronts of assault against my body. Give me the grace to implement the godly wisdom You are providing me, and help me to launch a counter-assault that will defeat prostate disease in my body forever. In Jesus' name, amen.

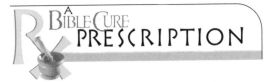

A BIBLE CURE PRESCRIPTION

What regular aerobic exercise are you now involved in?

_____

How often do you exercise?

_____

Are you willing to schedule exercise into your day as you would any other appointment?

_____

Outline your own personal exercise strategy.

_____

_____

Write a prayer in your own words asking for God's help to implement this fivefold strategic assault on your prostate disorder.

_____

_____

_____

Chapter 5

Succeeding Through Spirituality

By now you realize that God is not at all the weak and ineffective personality that He is often portrayed as being by our pop culture. The Bible portrays God as powerful, bold and a mighty victor in battle: "The LORD shall go forth like a mighty man; He shall stir up His zeal like a man of war. He shall cry out, yes, shout aloud; He shall prevail against His enemies," (Isa. 42:13, NKJV).

A vital key to accessing God's healing power is faith. God will prevail against His enemies of disease, and through exercising your faith, so will you. Let's take a look at faith and its dynamic link to God's healing power in you.

The Power of Faith

Faith is a mighty key to miracles. The Bible says that Jesus spoke to a tree that bore no fruit, and it withered and died. When the disciples asked about it, He taught them some valuable truths about faith.

> The disciples were amazed when they saw this and asked, "How did the fig tree wither so quickly?"
>
> Then Jesus told them, "I assure you, if you have faith and don't doubt, you can do things like this and much more. You can even say to this mountain, 'May God lift you up and throw you into the sea,' and it will happen. If you believe, you will receive whatever you ask for in prayer."
>
> —MATTHEW 21:20–22

This is an incredible promise. God Himself says to you that if you will simply believe, you can receive whatever you ask for from God. That's miracle-working power!

Faith for Your Complete Healing

The Bible says that nothing is impossible if you believe—including your healing from your prostate disorder. Once a deeply concerned father brought his little boy who had seizures to Jesus. He said, "If you can do anything, have compassion on

71

us and help us" (Mark 9:22, NKJV).

Jesus responded with a very powerful statement. He said, "If you can believe, all things are possible to him who believes" (v. 23, NKJV).

This caring father searched his own heart for an honest answer. Then he cried out, "Lord, I believe; help my unbelief!" (v. 24, NKJV).

In His statement, Christ handed this man a powerful key to accessing the healing power of God: belief,

> *And this is the victory that has overcome the world—our faith.*
> —1 JOHN 5:4, NAS

or faith. The man honestly said, "Yes, I really do believe." But the man had to admit that something else was stirring in his mind at the same time. In a moment the man asked Christ for help, saying, "Help my unbelief." Jesus answered both his requests because the child was instantly healed.

What about you? Do you believe but have to admit that questions and doubts arise in your mind as well? If so, do what this caring dad did. Turn your questions, doubts, problems and negative experiences about faith and healing over to God.

Most of us have had experiences that left us with negative feelings about faith. You've believed and were disappointed, or you know someone else who was deeply disappointed. You've heard preaching about faith or healing that turned you off. Perhaps you've just wondered if it's all fake or gimmickry.

Just give your doubts to God, and ask for His help with any unbelief you might have. I invite you to pray this prayer with me.

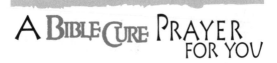

A BIBLE CURE PRAYER
FOR YOU

Dear Jesus Christ, I acknowledge that I often lack faith. I'm glad that You healed this man's boy despite his unbelief. I give You all of my unbelief and say with this caring father, "I do believe, but help my unbelief, too." I give You all of my doubts, negative thoughts and questions about healing. In Jesus' name, I ask You to strengthen my faith to believe and receive a healing for my prostate disorder. Amen.

Only for the Weak?

Some say faith is only for the weak, when actually it takes great strength and courage to believe. If you've ever endured a test of your faith, you know what I'm talking about. The Bible says that the greatest men in the world performed great acts of courage and feats of bravery because of their faith. It takes genuine guts to walk in faith.

The Bible records:

> It would take too long to recount the stories of the faith of Gideon, Barak, Samson, Jephthah, David, Samuel, and all the prophets. By faith these people overthrew kingdoms, ruled with justice, and received what God had promised them. They shut the mouths of lions, quenched the flames of fire, and escaped death by the edge of the sword. Their weakness was turned to strength. They became strong in battle and put whole armies to flight.
>
> —HEBREWS 11:32–34

Choose Faith

Some think that faith is a kind of mystical, eerie force that few people possess. Faith is not a force or a cloud or a mist or anything like that. Faith is nothing more than a bold, courageous decision to take God at His Word.

The Bible says that we've all been given a measure of faith. That means you have the faith you need to believe God to heal you. Give your doubts to God and keep believing—no matter what your circumstances tell you. That's the faith that moves mountains and sees the hand of God work miracles!

Now I challenge you to believe God to heal your body of prostate disease through the transcending power of faith. God is mightier than you could ever imagine, and His love for you is greater than your ability to comprehend. Trust Him today!

A BIBLE CURE PRAYER
FOR YOU

Heavenly Father, I thank You for Your amazing love for this friend of Yours who is reading this Bible Cure booklet. I pray for supernatural healing for him—for his body, mind and spirit. I thank You for Your amazing power to defeat disease in his body—not only that You have this power, but also that it is Your will to use it to defeat prostate disease in him. Help him employ the divine strategies You have provided for healing, prevention and divine health. Give him new, fresh strategies and insights for his life directly from Your throne. I pray that he would feel and experience Your amazing and wonderful love for him today and know without a doubt that You are real, You are alive, and You are his Father who cares deeply for him with a love that is beyond his ability to comprehend. In Jesus' mighty name, I agree with him in prayer for his healing. Amen.

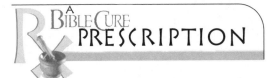

A BIBLE CURE PRESCRIPTION

Write a prayer asking God to heal your body of your prostate disorder.

_____

_____

_____

Write out your doubts and unbelief, and ask Him to help your unbelief.

_____

_____

_____

Write a bold declaration of your decision to choose faith.

_____

_____

_____

A Personal Note

From Don and Mary Colbert

God desires to heal you of disease. His Word is full of promises that confirm His love for you and His desire to give you His abundant life. His desire includes more than physical health for you; He wants to make you whole in your mind and spirit as well through a personal relationship with His Son, Jesus Christ.

If you haven't met my best friend, Jesus, I would like to take this opportunity to introduce Him to you. It is very simple.

If you are ready to let Him come into your heart and become your best friend, just bow your head and sincerely pray this prayer from your heart:

Lord Jesus, I want to know You as my Savior and Lord. I believe You are the Son of God and that You died for my sins. I also believe You were raised from the dead and now sit at the right hand of the Father praying for me. I ask You to forgive me for my sins and change my heart so that I can

*be Your child and live with You eternally.
Thank You for Your peace. Help me to
walk with You so that I can begin to know
You as my best friend and my Lord. Amen.*

If you have prayed this prayer, we rejoice with you in your decision and your new relationship with Jesus. Please contact us at pray4me@strang.com so that we can send you some materials that will help you become established in your relationship with the Lord. You have just made the most important decision of your life. We look forward to hearing from you.

Notes

CHAPTER 1
GAINING GROUND THROUGH UNDERSTANDING

1. Patrick Walsh, M.D. et al., *Dr. Patrick Walsh's Guide to Surviving Prostate Cancer* (New York: Warner Books, 2001).

CHAPTER 2
NEUTRALIZING SYMPTOMS THROUGH NUTRITION

1. J. Herbert et al., "Nutritional and Socioeconomic Factors in Relation to Prostate Cancer Mortality: A Cross-National Study," *Journal of the National Cancer Institute* 90, No. 21 (November 4, 1998): 1637–1647.

CHAPTER 4
ENERGIZING THROUGH EXERCISE,
ACTIVITIES AND TREATMENTS

1. For more information on Radiotherapy Clinics of Georgia, visit their website at www.rcog.net.
2. Source obtained from the Internet: Michael Smith, M.D., "PC-Spes Kills Cancer Cells, Stimulates the Immune System," *WebMD Medical News,* www.webMedHealth/prostate.
3. If you have prostate cancer, I recommend Dr. Patrick Walsh's book *Dr. Patrick Walsh's Guide to Surviving Prostate Cancer* (New York: Warner Books, 2001). If you, however, have metastatic prostate disease, I also recommend Dr. Jesse Stoff's book *The Prostate Miracle* (Kensington Publishing Corporation, 2000).

Ordering Information For Supplements

DIM (Indolplex)—800-931-1709

Divine Health Advanced Antioxidant—
407-331-7007

Divine Health Multivitamin for Men—
407-331-7007

Divine Health Prostate Support—
407-331-7007

Immuni-T—800-580-PLUS

Lycopene—Found in most health food
stores

MGW-3—Found in most health food
stores

Moducare—407-331-7007

Olive leaf extract—Found in most health
food stores

Don Colbert, M.D., was born in Tupelo, Mississippi. He attended Oral Roberts School of Medicine in Tulsa, Oklahoma, where he received a bachelor of science degree in biology in addition to his degree in medicine. Dr. Colbert completed his internship and residency with Florida Hospital in Orlando, Florida. He is board certified in family practice and has received extensive training in nutritional medicine.

If you would like more
information about natural and
divine healing, or information about
Divine Health Nutritional Products®,
you may contact
Dr. Colbert at:

1908 Boothe Circle
Longwood, FL 32750
Telephone: 407-331-7007
(for ordering products only)

Dr. Colbert's website is
www.drcolbert.com.

Disclaimer: Dr. Colbert and the staff of Divine Health Wellness Center are prohibited from addressing a patient's medical condition by phone, facsimile or e-mail. Please refer questions related to your medical condition to your own primary care physician.

Pick up these other Siloam Press
books by Dr. Colbert:

Toxic Relief
Walking in Divine Health
What You Don't Know May Be Killing You

The Bible Cure® Booklet Series

The Bible Cure for ADD and Hyperactivity
The Bible Cure for Allergies
The Bible Cure for Arthritis
The Bible Cure for Cancer
The Bible Cure for Candida and Yeast Infection
The Bible Cure for Chronic Fatigue and Fibromyalgia
The Bible Cure for Depression and Anxiety
The Bible Cure for Diabetes
The Bible Cure for Headaches
The Bible Cure for Heart Disease
The Bible Cure for Heartburn and Indigestion
The Bible Cure for High Blood Pressure
The Bible Cure for Irritable Bowel Syndrome
The Bible Cure for Memory Loss
The Bible Cure for Menopause
The Bible Cure for Osteoporosis
The Bible Cure for PMS and Mood Swings
The Bible Cure for Prostate Disorders
The Bible Cure for Sleep Disorders
The Bible Cure for Stress
The Bible Cure for Weight Loss and Muscle Gain

SILOAM PRESS

A part of Strang Communications Company
600 Rinehart Road
Lake Mary, FL 32746
(800) 599-5750